A Hospice Guide For Christians

"He Restores My Soul"

John Bridges

A Hospice Guide For Christians
"He Restores My Soul"
Copyright 2024 by John Bridges. All rights
reserved.
Published by The Souls Journey.
Published in the United States of America,
Series volume 1
Davisburg, MI.
Cover by J. Ruthenberg & Co.
Scripture quotations are from the New King James
Version®, Copyright ©1982 by Thomas Nelson: All
rights reserved.
ISBN: 979-8-9882803-0-9

In Remembrance of

Darlene
my wife, my love

Table of Contents

This Booklets Purpose

As a hospice spiritual care counselor (and having experience as a hospital chaplain and congregational pastor), I wrote and provided this hospice booklet for my patients, their families, and hospice staff.

In my experience, I've observed that when someone discovers they have six months or less to live, several responses can be triggered:

- Christians will seek affirmation, reaffirmation, and comfort in their relationship with God and others.

- Emotional pain is often experienced, associated with anticipatory grief with four distinctive feelings of loss.

- Christians want biblical guidance during emotional pain associated with anticipatory grief.

- Patients and families seek information about end-of-life physical changes. They also seek information about what to do during the dying one's last hours, including **things not to do.**

This booklet's section headings often become discussion starters for patients' and families' particular needs.

This booklet is also an excellent resource guide for congregational care.

Affirming Our Faith

Life is like a train ride, with people getting on and others getting off at every stop. You may be reading this booklet because life for someone close to you is ending.

Where is God for us in all of this? As Christians, we affirm that the message of the cross of Jesus Christ holds the answer. Stay focused on the message, affirming and reaffirming your faith.

Examples of spiritual affirmation throughout life:

- Your pastor asks affirmation questions before a baptism.

- Holy Communion brings us to a place of self-examination and reaffirmation (1 Corinthians 11:28).

- Anointing (as with prayer for the sick, James 5:13-16) also brings us to a place of reflection, affirmation, and confession.

- Praying the Lord's Prayer refocuses our relationship with God and others.

- Singing the hymns and spiritual songs of the church provides assurance and reconfirmation.

For Christians, our spiritual journey starts and ends with trusting in the resurrected Jesus because He died for our sins on the cross. Brothers and sisters, come to the cross with me (by way of a short devotional), and let us affirm and reaffirm our faith in Jesus.

A Christian Devotional

They Looked, and They Lived, An Ancient Cure for Snakebite (Numbers 21:4-9 and John 3:14-16)

Moses was the leader of a mass migration. After 400 years of slavery, several million Jews were set free by God's Passover miracle, and they were going home to the Promised Land.

The Jews became discouraged during their long journey through the desert because they were hot, thirsty, and tired of the food supplied by God.

That's when they made a bad mistake.

They started complaining against God (who protected them) and against their leader, Moses. God sent poisonous snakes into the camp; many people were bitten and died. "Therefore the people came to Moses and said, 'We have sinned, for we have spoken against the LORD and you; pray to the LORD that He take away the snakes from us.' So Moses prayed for the people" (Numbers 21:5-7).

God told Moses to make a snake out of bronze, then put the bronze snake on a pole and lift it high in the air. And God said, "It shall be that everyone who is bitten when he looks at it, shall live" (21:8). And God's servant obeyed. "Moses made a bronze serpent, and put it on a pole; and so it was if a serpent had bitten anyone when he looked at the bronze serpent, he lived" (21:9).

Imagine our being there with Moses about 3,400 years ago—discouraged, rebellious, snake-bitten, and dying in the hot desert. Then we confess our sins and look at God's only cure for our snakebite. Immediately we're forgiven and cured! And we worship God.

Now imagine you and me sitting in a house with Jesus, some 1,400 years after Moses. We see and hear Jesus teaching a man how to trust God and receive forgiveness.

3

Attentively, we listen as Jesus says this:

> "And as Moses lifted up the serpent in the wilderness, even so, must the son of Man be lifted up, that whoever believes in Him should not perish but have eternal life. For God so loved the world that He gave His only begotten Son, that whoever believes in Him should not perish but have everlasting life". (John 3:14-16)

God provided the **antidote** for snakebite—physically healing those who looked at the brass snake, which Moses lifted up.

God also provided the **antidote** for sin—the spiritual healing that comes from the forgiveness of sins for those trusting in Jesus, who was crucified, died, was buried, and rose from the dead.

God says, **"Believe!"** And His Word testifies of Jesus, "To Him, all the prophets witness that, through His name, whoever believes in Him will receive remission of sins" (Acts 10:43).

* * *

Forgiven?

Some are unsure that their sins have been forgiven.

To reaffirm—or to become sure of—your forgiveness in Christ, I invite you to pray this prayer between you and God:

> God, I come to you **in the name of Jesus.** The snake-bit Jews believed what You said and looked at the bronze snake for healing. I believe Jesus was crucified, that He died for my sins and was buried, and that He rose from the grave—and that whoever looks to Him for the forgiveness of sin is forgiven. I look, I believe, and I call to you, God, forgive me in Jesus's name—and I live! Thank you for your forgiveness![*]

---

[*] "You can know for sure you will go to heaven," https://peacewithgod.net/steps/; accessed 4-20-24

4

Your Pastor and Hospice Chaplain can help you in many ways, including these:

- Collaborating with you to develop a plan of care that meets your spiritual needs.
- Increasing a sense of security for the patient and family by encouraging the expression of love and forgiveness.
- Assisting in the resolution of unresolved issues.
- Decreasing fear and anxiety regarding death and the dying process.
- Explaining the causes of spiritual and emotional pain for a dying person and family.
- Discussing and explaining the key sources and types of grief.
- Facilitating discussion of decline toward the end of life.
- Provide or arrange for pastoral services in your church, such as anointing the sick, reconciliation, communion, or baptism.
- Encourage discussion about planning a meaningful funeral or memorial service.
- The hospice chaplain will meet you where you are and has <u>no agenda</u> to change you.
- The Hospice Chaplain <u>will not</u> attempt to take your pastor's place.

  Suppose a hospice patient refuses pastoral care. In that case, the pastoral care person will not impose themselves on the patient. But (if acceptable to the family), they will gladly meet with any family member separately.

Causes of Spiritual Pain

Hospice patients and their families may experience spiritual pain and suffering. Spiritual pain can result from uncertain or broken relationships with God or others. Restored friendship with God and others can bring **feelings of spiritual peace.**

Here are some specific causes of spiritual pain.

Uncertainty That God Will Forgive

A patient (with the initials B.B.) had spiritual pain and suffering from his uncertainty that God would forgive him. He'd dropped out of the church as a young man and now was old and dying. Like some, B.B. thought he wasn't good enough to ask God for forgiveness; he was unaware that Jesus accepts all who genuinely come to Him.

What does God's Word say about forgiveness? In Acts 10:43, the apostle Peter proclaimed this about Jesus: "To Him all the prophets witness that, through His name, whoever believes in Him will receive remission of sins." My patient, B.B., believed the promise of forgiveness found throughout Scripture; he confessed to God and received forgiveness and spiritual peace. I saw the sincerity in his restoration when he said, "I'll have my son take me to church, so I can tell them *I'm back!*"

(Suggested Scripture readings: John 3:14-16; 1 John 1:9; Matthew 11:28-30.)

Lack of Forgiveness Toward Others

"I hate him and don't want to forgive him!"

Perhaps your wounded heart says, "I cannot forgive." But your loving Savior Jesus says, "If you do not forgive others their trespasses, neither will your Father forgive your trespasses" (Matthew 6:15).

A fellow worker, Jim, did not like Bill and continually found ways to insult him, refusing reconciliation. This situation would confront Bill every time he prayed. Bill told God, "I hate Jim and don't want to forgive him!" After struggling with his emotions, Bill said, "Okay, God, I'll do what you say and forgive him—regardless of how I feel." For two weeks, in his morning prayers, Bill would say, "I forgive Jim for his actions."

Then a miracle happened! One morning, as Bill prayed, he realized he no longer hated Jim. Jim never changed, but Bill experienced spiritual healing.

It may take time for our emotions to catch up with God's reality! (For further reading on how often to forgive another, see Matthew 18:21-22.)

Putting Off Making Things Right

"I'll make him suffer; I refuse to forgive him until tomorrow!"

Lea's father-in-law Abe had apologized for offending her. But she decided to withhold forgiveness and make him suffer for a while; she planned to accept his apology the next day. But that night, the Nazi death squad took Abe away and shot him.

(For further reading on Jesus's teaching on the urgency of reconciliation with others, see Matthew 5:23 and Luke 11:4.)

"Be angry, and do not sin: do not let the sun go down on your wrath, nor give place to the devil" (Ephesians 4:26).

My friend Dr. Ten Robertson (a hospice spiritual care counselor) often counsels his clients, "Face it *today!*"

Living in Victimville

Corrie ten Boom ran a home for World War II survivors of Nazi prison camps. Corrie said, "Those who were able to forgive their former enemies were also able to return to the outside world and rebuild their lives, no matter the physical scars. Those who nursed their bitterness remained invalids. It was as simple and as horrible as that."[*]

If others have asked you for forgiveness, they are now free of moral guilt as far as God is concerned. And even if they have not requested your forgiveness (and refuse to talk with you, you are still required to forgive them (If only between you and God).

(On forgiving others, see Matthew 18:21-35.)

Remember, Forgiving Others is Not About Feelings. It is About Obeying God!

If we're withholding forgiveness...

- We are *not* punishing the offender but only destroying ourselves.
- We're sinning against God.
- We're trapped in Victimville because we refuse to do what is right: to forgive someone else.

(For further reading: Philippians 4:13; Ephesians 4:32; Luke 23:34.)

False Guilt

A Christian may say, "I can't forgive myself! This statement needs to be examined and clarified.by biblical standards of guilt. "

---

[*] Corrie ten Boom, in "Guideposts Classics: Corrie ten Boom on Forgiveness," https://guideposts.org/positive-living/guideposts-classics- corrie-ten-boom-forgiveness/; accessed November 1, 2022.

Are you experiencing false guilt?

Answer each of the following four questions Yes or No:

1. Have I personally trusted Jesus to forgive me? *(See page 4)*

2. Have I confessed known sins to God in Jesus' name?

3. If needful, have I asked others for forgiveness?

4. If needful, have I forgiven others?

Christians who can say "yes" to questions 1-4 and are still feeling guilty may feel personal embarrassment, regret, and disappointment. You may be having feelings of *false guilt.* God has pronounced you forgiven, so redirect your thoughts and life to the now and the future. False guilt will try to capture you again, so revisit this booklet section until God's grace reality replaces your feelings of false guilt.

How did the Apostle Paul deal with his past? Listen to his words:

> But one thing I do, forgetting those things which are behind and reaching forward to those things which are ahead, I press on toward the goal to win the prize for which God has called me heavenward in Christ Jesus. (Philippians 3:13-14).

If false guilt feelings are persistent, you may be dealing with emotional pain. Meet for pastoral counseling and consult your physician to eliminate physical reasons for these feelings.

Understanding and receiving reconciliation with God and others are essential to spiritual peace. *Reconciliation removes spiritual pain.*

The Feelings Behind Emotional Pain

Grief is the natural response to loss. (Your hospice team has grief support personnel and literature available to you, so I will limit my grief discussion here.)

Emotional pain is a natural response to *grief*—and may not be connected to spiritual pain.

- **Anticipatory grief** is when we know death will occur and feel (at some level) as if it has already happened.

- **Compound grief** is when we have multiple losses close together.

- **Disinfranchised grief** is grief that isn't acknowledged as legitimate or is overlooked by others around us. For example, a loss may be seen (by others) as too small or the relationship too distant to justify grieving. (Don't overlook—and thus minimize—the grief of young and early adolescent children. Your hospice agency has literature to help children who are grieving.)

We grieve as groups, as families, and most importantly, as individuals—because everyone's grief is theirs. And there's no set schedule for grief. Feelings of denial, anger, bargaining, depression, and acceptance will come and go as they will.

Actress Amanda Blake once said, "Tears are not the measure of grief."

Let's unravel and examine the *feelings* of 1) loss of control, 2) loss of purpose, 3) loss of relationships, and 4) loss of self. These four are part of your emotional pain. These feelings of loss are like a cord of four strings; each is alive, always intermingling with the other senses of loss. It will be helpful to unravel this cord and discuss which loss is dominating your feelings at any time.[*]

Understanding Our Feelings of Loss as Death Approaches

As children, we all had dreams and aspirations of what we would be growing up. Peer approval is essential to most; our self-image is connected to our relationships. This connectedness influences our life purpose and our need to find and maintain some measure of control.

Let's look closer at these four feelings of loss.

Feelings Regarding Loss of Control

"You'll get my Harley keys when you pry them from my cold, stiff hands!"

Your possessions and physical abilities have been an extension of yourself. You were in control, but that is changing. You may have prayed, "God, how can I cope with these losses? I need a miracle!"

God can give us peace, which will sustain us through feelings of loss of control. Listen to His instruction as well as His promise about this:

> Be anxious for nothing, but in everything by prayer and supplication, with thanksgiving, let your requests be made known to God; and the peace of God, which surpasses all understanding, will guard your hearts and minds through Christ Jesus. (Philippians 4:6-7)

---

[*] Chaplain Dick Millspaugh, "The God Understands Series"; American Bible Society; https://neveralonemilitary.com/, accessed September 5, 2022.

Feelings Regarding Loss of Relationships

When was the first time God said something was not good?

Here it is: "And the LORD God said, "*It is* not good that man should be alone; I will make him a helper comparable to him" (Genesis 2:18).

God created us as relational beings. The Scriptures remind us of our eternal relationship with other Christians and with God.

Here's a description in God's Word of those in heaven:

> But ye are come unto mount Sion, and unto the city of the living God, the heavenly Jerusalem, and to an innumerable company of angels, to the general assembly and church of the firstborn, which are written in heaven, and to God the Judge of all, and to the spirits of just men made perfect, and to Jesus the mediator of the new covenant. (Hebrews 12:23)

Feelings Regarding Loss of Purpose

"Why am I still here?"

The Scriptures encourage us regarding our eternal destination and our need to complete this life's purpose. Providing care to hospice patients often includes facilitating life review. These times of life reviews can be significant for patients who reflect upon and search for the deeper meaning of their lives.

Regarding purpose, God's Word tells us, "To everything there is a season, a time for every purpose under heaven: a time to be born, and a time to die..." (Ecclesiastes 3:1-2).

The apostle Paul wrote the following just before his death as a martyr:

The time of my departure is at hand. I have fought the good fight, I have finished the race, I have kept the faith. Finally, there is laid up for me the crown of righteousness, which the Lord, the righteous Judge, will give to me on that day, and not to me only but also to all who have loved His appearing. (2 Timothy 4:6-8).

Rites of passage* are significant, so if possible, involve the hospice patient in planning his or her funeral.

Feelings Regarding Loss of Self

"I've been Sally, the hairdresser, for most of my life. Who am I going to be when I die?"

Self-identity is about who we were and who we are, and it reaches into the future, asking, *Who will I be in the afterlife?*

God speaks to us in answer:

Beloved, *now* we are children of God, and it has not yet been revealed what we shall be, but we know that when He is revealed, *we shall be like Him*, for we shall see Him as He is. (1 John 3:2)

Jesus sees these feelings of loss of control, loss of relationships, loss of purpose, and loss of self—and He provides us with spiritual strength from these sources:

- The Holy Bible (see Psalm 119:11-12).
- The Holy Spirit lives within all who have trusted Jesus Christ (see John 3:14-16; 7:37-39).
- Our family (physical and spiritual), supporting and affirming us (see Hebrews 10:24-25).

---

* Rite of Passage: A ceremony or series of ceremonies, often very ritualized, to celebrate a transition in a person's life. Baptisms, mitzvahs, weddings, and funerals are among the best-known examples. The American Heritage® Dictionary of the English Language, 5th Edition.

Biblical Response to Emotional Pain

Feeling Sorrowful Without Complaining Sinfully[*]

Did you know that there are sorrowful psalms?

Every psalm is not a happy-clappy psalm. 53 out of 150 are psalms of crying or sorrow in Psalms. They say things like, "God, where are you?"

They say, *God, it seems like you are silent. God, it looks like you have abandoned us.* They're honest, and they're speaking to God. *God, it seems the wicked are doing better than we are.*

Christianity is not about acting. So, the psalms of lamentation permit us to acknowledge these emotions. (One example is Psalm 142.)

Christians need to understand that God doesn't expect us to pretend. "I know what I ought to think and be; I just need to pretend I'm always there." When you're *not* there—and you know you're not—the question is, "What do I do with this?" Well, there are 53 Psalms for that, the Psalms of lamentation.

Overcoming a Complaining Spirit

How can I prevent myself from slipping into sinful complaining, or how can I help myself out of that state if I'm already there?

I've found three things helpful in my life as I point others in this direction.

- *Submit* to the authority of God. Pray as Jesus prayed, "Thy will be done" (Matthew 6:10)

---

[*] From the blog post "Being Sorrowful Without Complaining Sinfully" by Brad Bigney, lead pastor at Grace Fellowship Church in Florence, Kentucky, and a certified biblical counselor with ACBC; https://biblicalcounseling.com/resource-library/conference-messages/biblical-sorrow-without-sinful-complaining/; edited and used with permission.

- *Spend time* with those who love God and joyfully serve others. "Finally, all of you be of one mind, having compassion for one another; love as brothers, be tenderhearted, be courteous." (1 Peter 3:8)
- *Listen and consider* what God says about eternity: "For the things which are seen are temporary, but the things which are not seen are eternal" (2 Corinthians 4:18).

As I've reflected on what Scripture says in 1 Corinthians 15:50-58 about our final victory over death, I've concluded: **Grief is the unwanted guest who visits every person, attempting to preoccupy our present with the unchangeable past or future. *Grief must not become our master.* Hope in the resurrection is our master.**

Keeping Up the Humor

"A joyful heart is good medicine" (Proverbs 17:22).

Grandpa Joe was a hospice patient, often visited by his grandchildren. Five-year-old Sally would play make-believe games with Joe. One afternoon, she said,

"Let's play frog, Grandpa."

Grandpa said, "Okay, what do you want me to do?'

"You just need to croak like a frog because Cousin Jack said, "After Grandpa croaks, we'll go on vacation!" Grandpa laughed and laughed, later telling everyone the story. After that, he greeted all his friends and family with a croak…until the day he cr—!

Fear of The Unknown
"Doctor, I'm Afraid to Die"*

A sick man turned to his doctor as he prepared to leave the examination room and said, "Doctor, I'm afraid to die. Tell me what lies on the other side."

Very quietly, the doctor said, "I don't know."

"You don't? You—a Christian man—don't know what's on the other side?"

The doctor was holding the door handle. From the door's other side came the sound of scratching and whining. As he opened the door, a dog sprang into the room and leaped on him with an eager show of gladness.

Turning to the patient, the doctor said, "Did you notice my dog? He's never been in this room before. He didn't know what was inside. He knew nothing except that his master was here, and when the door opened, he sprang in without fear." Then he said, "To answer your question, I know little of what's on the other side. But I know my Master Jesus Christ is there, and that's enough."

---

* Quoted from the Cybersalt website, www.cybersalt.org/illustrations/fear-of-death; author unknown. Accessed Sept.6, 2022

As a chaplain, I encourage you to draw strength from:

- God using the resources of Scripture
- Your family and friends
- Your pastor and your spiritual care counselor.

Meanwhile, the remaining chapters here deal with end-of-life signs and symptoms that hospice patients and families may expect (although not all of these signs may be present).

Signs of Distress*

Emotional Signs

- Anger
- Denial of illness or the reality of the prognosis
- Depression, feeling "flat"
- Troubling dreams, nightmares
- Fear
- Feeling of powerlessness and loss of control
- Restlessness, agitation, anxiety

Behavioral Signs

- Active forms of self-harm
- Frantic searching for advice from everyone
- Turning away from former religious practice and affiliation, refusing visits from religious leaders
- Lack of engagement with activities meant to bring comfort or joy
- Metaphorical or symbolic language suggesting distress or unresolved concerns
- Power struggles with caregivers or family
- Putting oneself in an unsafe position
- Asking "Why?" or questioning the duration of the dying process

---

* Information on pages 23-26 includes common medical knowledge. Many hospice websites post various forms of this information.

- Refusing assistance in personal care
- Refusing to take pain medication
- Speaking about "not wanting to be a burden."
- Struggling in various ways over the loss of independence
- Experiencing conflict between the goals of palliative care and religious beliefs
- Fixation on nutrition, herbal remedies, or looking for a miraculous cure
- Withdrawal, isolation

Physical Signs

- Shortness of breath
- Sleeplessness
- Unrelieved pain sometimes is of a spiritual or emotional source.

Postponing Pastoral Care Until The Last Hours Is Unwise Because:

- Some hospice patients have unresolved fears and questions which require multiple sessions.

- Many patients won't be alert enough to verbalize their heartfelt needs during their last hours.

- Everyone's death is unique. Only God knows when someone will die, so it's best not to delay or put off visits by a pastor, family, and friends.

Signs of Dying

Pre-Active Phase of Dying

- Apnea—periods where breathing stops for several seconds before starting again, either while awake or while sleeping
- Edema—the swelling of the body or extremities with fluid
- Restlessness (resulting from increased anxiety), the inability to get comfortable, confusion, agitation, and nervousness
- Increased inability to heal from bruises, infections, or wounds
- Increased periods of inactivity, lethargy, or sleep
- Loss of interest in daily activities
- Loss of interest in eating or drinking
- Statements about seeing people who are already dead
- Putting one's "ducks in order," making amends, or catching up while talking to family and friends
- "Tying up loose ends" in concern over finances—wills, trusts, insurance
- Statements about dying soon or asking questions about death
- Withdrawal from social activities, with more time spent alone or at home

Active Phase of Dying

- A continued drop in blood pressure to 20 to 30 points below average; a systolic pressure below 70, with a diastolic below 50

- Decrease in urination, with urine darkening in color or changing colors

- Difficulties swallowing liquids or resistance to all food and drink

- Increased difficulty waking from sleep

- Mottling of the arms, legs, hands, and feet, giving a blue or purple splotchy appearance to the skin

- Possible loss of hearing, feeling, smell, taste, or sight at the final stage

- Possible marked changes in personality, acting wildly; severe agitation or hallucinations

- Significant changes in breathing; congestion, a buildup of fluid in the lungs

- More extended periods of apnea and abnormal breathing patterns, such as cycles of slow then fast breathing

- Sleep so deep that they can't be aroused; a coma-like state

- Not moving for long periods

- Unresponsiveness; inability to speak

- Stating, "I am going to die soon."

- Hands, feet, arms, and legs become very cold to the touch

- Stating that they're numb or cannot feel anything

- Urinary or bowel incontinence

Preparing for the Last Hours

Provide a Comfortable Environment

Calmness and gentleness in our voices toward the person dying can comfort them and help them feel less afraid or alone. The dying can often sense people in the room or hear you speaking to them right up to the end. Some patients have someone sitting beside them, gently holding a hand. Some like to listen to words of comfort from Scripture. Calming, gentle music will set a peaceful atmosphere.

Friends and family members can take turns being present so no one gets overly tired. Take breaks occasionally (with the patient's permission), giving your loved one private personal time.

The caregivers should provide a clean, well-ventilated, and temperature-controlled room where loving, caring friends, family, and pets are welcome.

Things *Not* to Do During Your Loved One's Last Hours[*]

I've witnessed many families struggling because they don't know what to do during the last hours of a person's life. Many people lack knowledge and have misconceptions about a dying person's needs as they approach the end. Here are guidelines on what to avoid.

---

[*] Adapted from Manteau-Rao, "In the End: "10 Things Not to Do During a Loved One's Last Hours," "https://www.huffpost.com/entry/hospice- death_b_850216, accessed Sept.6, 2022; used by permission.

Do *not* insist on feeding the person.

We're so used to equating caring with nurturing with food. As the body shuts down, the requirements for food progressively stop, and it becomes essential not to get in the way of this process. We need to shift our view of what's normal to make room for the reality of the dying one.

Do not give the person a drink.

As with food, the dying one's ability to take in liquids stops, and it becomes necessary not to force water intake.

Do not interfere with prescribed pain medication for your loved one.

Your loved one's comfort is at stake. Respect the hospice team's decision regarding which and how much pain medications to give. If it looks like your loved one is still in pain, signal it to the nurse in charge and explore ways to increase comfort.

Do not talk about the person as if they aren't present.

Provide the right atmosphere for the death experience. Again, be aware that the dying can often sense people in the room or hear you speaking to them right up to the end. Talking to the person dying can comfort them and help them feel less afraid or alone.

Suppose the person appears unresponsive or speaks in a way that does not make sense; refrain from talking in the third person about them. D.o not share information that could be upsetting or disrespectful to the dying.

Don't shut the dying person out of the family conversation.

Include him or her as a natural part of the ongoing room conversations with *statements that don't require an answer*. An example might be, "Jill, I remember when you took me to the amusement park." You then tell your experience with Jill and the fun you had.

Do not argue with the patient.

In cases when the person becomes restless and wants to get out of bed, do not argue. Instead, reassure them with a calm voice and decrease any unnecessary stimulation that could increase restlessness. Holding the patient's hand (without rubbing) may also help lessen the agitation.

Keep the atmosphere pleasant. No arguing allowed! Do *not* fight with other family members in the patient's room.

While sometimes unavoidable, such quarrels create unnecessary distress for the dying person. Advocate for the patient and ask your family to discuss such matters elsewhere.

Do *not* be surprised by the look and sound of death.

Be prepared for changes in how the person breathes, interacts, feels, and looks. The death rattle can be scary if you've never witnessed it before. Immediately call the "On call" or your hospice R.N. regarding changes in breathing patterns or rattle so she can make medication adjustments if needed.

The dying person may have tearing, half-open, glassy eyes and the touch of a stiff, cold body. *You need to know that these are not painful but typical physical manifestations of near death.*

Do *not* shake the person into returning to life when they stop breathing.

I've often watched relatives try to shake their dying loved ones out of the immobility of impending death. While you may be unable to accept the reality of the imminent passing of your loved one, you must respect the fact of it.

Do *not* get agitated around the person.

Hold each other accountable! If necessary, leave the room to recompose yourself. One natural response to seeing a loved one dying is becoming anxious and talking nervously or loudly when we should be quiet. Such a display of anxiety upsets the dying person and adds to their distress. Instead, calm yourself and bring the gift of your quiet presence to your loved one.

Remember, this is not about *doing* for the person but *being with* him or her. Read them a favorite scripture or poem. Hold their hand.

Do *not* move the hospice patient back to the hospital without first calling and *consulting with* the hospice R.N. case manager or the on-call R.N. Please *ask your hospice R.N. the reasons for this warning!*

Caring for your loved one in a crisis means calling the R.N. case manager or after-hours nurse and doing what they say! They've already seen every kind of situation that you and your loved one will face.

And remember, your hospice team will know what action plan will be best for your loved one during a crisis. Your hospice team is available 24/7 and only a phone call away.

The hospice care team's goal is the same as your goal— to let your loved one die naturally and in peace.

The Caregiver's Self-Care:

- Accept your loved one's imminent death because your current role is to be calm, comforting, and present.
- Take care of yourself. Get some sleep, eat something, pray, take a walk, and share your grief and caregiving with others.
- Caregivers can break themselves physically and emotionally by refusing help!

"Now, the God of peace be with you all. Amen." (Romans 15:33)

* * *

The Lord's Prayer

Our Father who art in heaven
Hollowed be Thy name

Thy kingdom come

Thy will be done
On earth, as it is in heaven

Give us this day our daily bread

And forgive us our sins, as we forgive
those who sin against us

Lead us not into temptation, but deliver us
from evil

For Thine is the kingdom, and the power,
and the glory forever

Amen

About the Author

John Bridges and his late wife, Darlene, were married for fifty-four years. They have an awesome daughter, Rebecca (married to Marc), three granddaughters, and two beautiful great-granddaughters.

John has many fond memories of his late family members, including his wife Darlene, son Adam, daughter-in-law Jennifer, and grandson John.

He earned his M.A. in New Testament Studies from Ashland Theological Seminary. He completed a two-year (post-graduate) CPE Residency at William Beaumont Hospital in Royal Oak, Michigan.

John has ministered as a pastor, a hospice spiritual care counselor, a chaplain, and a minister of Christian education.

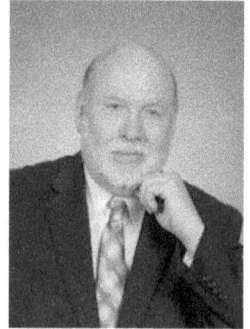

johnabridges.com